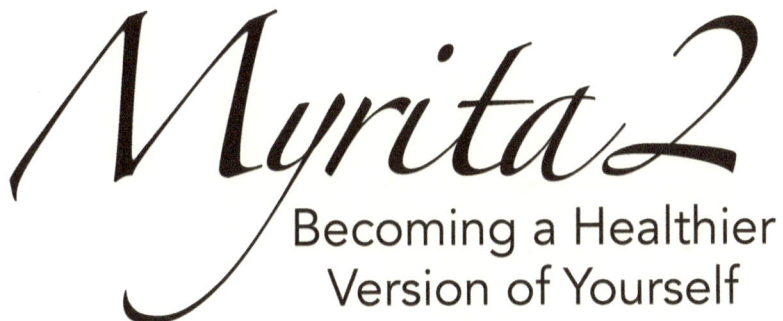

Becoming a Healthier
Version of Yourself

Louise YT Phua

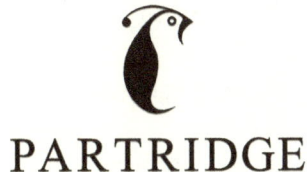

PARTRIDGE

Illustration by Sophia Yong

Print information available on the last page.

To order additional copies of this book, contact
Toll Free +65 3165 7531 (Singapore)
Toll Free +60 3 3099 4412 (Malaysia)
orders.singapore@partridgepublishing.com

www.partridgepublishing.com/singapore

I dedicate *Myrita2* to every earthling who
has survived the COVID-19 pandemic.
Hopefully, we have learnt important lessons
to better care and appreciate ourselves,
our communities, and Mother Earth.
I believe when we grasp collectively with panic as a human
race, there is hope for an exhale into a brighter future.

- Louise YT Phua

*Let food be thy medicine
and medicine be thy food.
- Hippocrates, Greek physician*

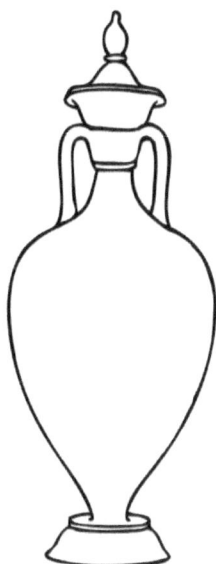

Contents

PART C: MORE USEFUL HEALTH TIPS

Disclaimer

Myrita2 comprises of guidelines and health tips that the author lives by. They are by no means definitive medical solution for every ailment.

Myrita2 does not purport to be a cure-all for any illness or disease. This booklet provides general information only. It is not a substitute for professional medical advice. Readers with existing medical conditions ought to seek professional advice for appropriate diet and nutritional intake.

Food fads come and go, while some food traditions persist for centuries. Do not overconsume certain foods for specific benefits. All things in moderation.

To support self-directed earthlings to integrate more nourishing plant-based products into their daily meals, *Myrita2* is written for the novice home cooks who aspire to be slightly healthier versions of themselves.

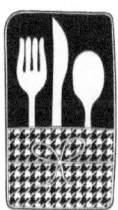

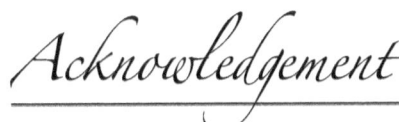

Acknowledgement

Our family is blessed to consult with highly qualified medical professionals, including Dr and Mrs Kenneth Chiew, Dr Wu Xiao Siew (Beijing Tong Ren Tang), Dr Yue Bao Sheng (master acupuncturist), Dr David Wu Wei Hua (previously practising neurosurgeon), Dr Ong Mei Hong (food scientist), and Dr and Mrs Huang Zhong Yi (retired internal medicine physicians). We are grateful for the many years of medical care from you. Your tips on rainbow diet and clean eating have guided our wellness and well-being for decades.

Several domestic goddesses are key influencers of my healthy lifestyle - my paternal grandmother, my maternal grandmother, my mother, Aunty Hong, Aunty Ivy, and Aunty Lian Zhu. None of these domestic goddesses believe in ultraprocessed foods. In the fashion of the slow food movement, most of our mothers rely on fresh local produce to whip up mouth-watering dishes. Often, you cook our family meals from scratch with fresh ingredients. At home, you rarely allow us to eat packaged foods. Thanks to the influence of my domestic goddesses, I declare I am a bland food queen.

Tan See Yang, my favourite big brother, with every good intention, you constantly cast your watchful eyes over my shoulders.

Joseph Wong, my book mentor, for both my publications, you play a critical role in shaping the contents and development. I am grateful for your astute command.

Sophia Yong, founder and owner of National Accounting and a business consultant on systems and efficient operations in finance, you are a living example of having a holistic approach in health and beauty. You firmly believe in keeping the child in us alive and that adults can continue to doodle and splatter colourful paints. As the chief illustrator for *Myrita2*, your commitment to your artistic development is admirable.

My eco-conscious friends and green activists Gobbs Lim Siew Yuen, Foo Piao Xu, Debbie Han, and Gan Geok Joo, your pursuit of all things natural and organic is phenomenal. I appreciate trading tips on vegetable gardening and health matters with all of you.

Lala Olga Wagner, German- born and Russian-raised, banking and robotics specialist, passionate dancer and diver, your keen interest in Asian cuisine is inspiring. Meanwhile, I am looking forward to more fusion recipes from you (see page 33).

And you, the readers, your feedback and support are immensely encouraging. I remain motivated and committed to make my *Myrita* series even better for you.

Stay tuned.

With gratitude,
Louise YT Phua

Prologue

Life is a balancing act. Finding the right balance is a constant challenge.

Technologies continue to innovate the way food is grown, harvested, processed, transported, and consumed. A wide array of food products is now available to the urban masses. Given the busy urban lifestyle, how many of us have taken the time to pause and ponder about what we are eating? How have we prospered from the large array of ultraprocessed foods that is easily available?

More and more, we are constantly connected to our digital devices. How often do we pay attention to our physical activities and exercise regimes? Have we pondered about our fixation on instant gratification and miracle cures?

The Wake-Up Calls

In recent years, several coaching clients I encountered gave me these wake-up calls:

Linn, thirty-seven, was a highly sought-after award-winning web designer. At the height of her stellar career, she took the top trophy at a global design contest. Often, Linn stared at her desktop for fourteen straight hours to produce the finest artwork that wowed the most demanding clients. A chronic insomniac, She lived on frozen meals during most of her workdays. One thunderous afternoon, she fainted in a taxi queue while travelling to a client meeting. At the hospital where she was admitted, Linn was diagnosed with lupus. Lupus is an autoimmune disease that attacks the joints and the organs. For almost six months, she lived in shock. Linn could not accept that her health was in dire state. She took a two-year sabbatical at a Balinese fruit farm to tend to her ill health and slowly recuperated.

Tian was appointed country manager of a Scandinavian shipping company when she was twenty-eight. Every evening, she was scheduled for multiple dinner parties at lavish restaurants. Her life revolved around wining and dining with high-level government officials and business owners in the transportation sector, so as to court multimillion-dollar deals. Before the age of forty, she launched three profitable businesses, acquired seven properties, and possessed a suite of luxury cars. Reluctantly, Tian had to undergo a health check due to an insurance requirement. Her worst nightmare came true when the health check revealed that she had fatty liver. When her liver accumulated excessive fat, it malfunctioned and triggered a host of health problems. On her forty-fifth birthday, her fatty liver was at the verge of collapse. Tian was devastated and went into seclusion.

Kelly was a rising star in the pharmaceuticals industry. At forty-two, he headed the Asia-Pacific region of a major healthcare conglomerate. Originally from a small town in Massachusetts, USA, Kelly was a mediocre college student. Intrigued by Asian culture, He got himself a job stint in southeast China upon graduation. For over two decades, the workaholic built his career in one of the world's fastest growing economies. On a daily basis, Kelly drank several cans of carbonated drinks and beer. During the weekends, he ate seven hamburgers at one go and was twenty kilogrammes overweight. Kelly had little physical activities. In less than a year of his rapid promotion, he died of a sudden heart attack during a business trip to north China.

These corporate citizens are high achievers with one thing in common. That is, their stellar careers came to a standstill due to their poor health. Their poor health were the outcomes of neglect and oversight. During their younger days, they took their health for granted and were lulled into the false assumption of being invincible. Until bad news struck.

Poor health arises from poor immunity. Immunity is protection from diseases. For those of us who live busy urban lifestyles, we now have easy access to a wide variety of instant gratification, including fast food, carbonated drinks, frozen meals, and microwavable items. Knowingly or unknowingly, the instant gratification may potentially harm our health in the long term. According to WebMD (2020), twelve factors suppress our immunity, which subsequently lead to poor health. These factors include high-fat diet, alcohol, too few fruits and vegetables, lack of essential vitamins and minerals, no sex, smoking, too little time outdoors, grief, anxiety, certain medications, lack of sleep, and lack of exercise.

I, too, was not spared. For several years, I was plagued by constant outbreak of eczema and skin rashes. My hands, inside elbows, back of knees, and neck would be covered with large patches of itchy little bumps. Several visits to the dermatologists did not resolve my skin problem. The embarrassment and frustration adversely affected my emotional and mental well-being.

I researched medical news on eczema. I observed and studied my own diet and lifestyle. I read widely about food and nutrition, gut health, and life changes. Advocates of clean eating and slow food movement are vocal about the overuse of chemical substances in industrial farming methods and factory-processed food. Subsequently, I cut down most ultraprocessed foods from my diet. Additionally, I watched my stress level and eliminated fragrance from cosmetics and toilets. Gradually, my skin recovered.

The Significance of Teochew Eating Habits

I am blessed to be born into a Teochew family. Before World War II, my grandparents migrated from Guangdong Province in south China in search of a better life for the family in Singapore.

With no exposure to other cultures, my paternal grandmother only knew how to cook Teochew dishes. Southeast Asian ingredients such as *sambal belacan* (chilli sauce), *pandan* (screw pine leaves), aloe vera, and nutmeg were unknown to her. Often, our family meals were painstakingly prepared from scratch. Ultraprocessed foods were not in her grocery shopping baskets. Her daughters, daughters-in-law, and subsequently granddaughters and great-granddaughters follow many of her culinary practices. Likewise, the male members of our family are supportive of clean eating.

Most of our family members live on diets with low sugar, low salt, and little oil. We favour the natural taste of fresh produce. Traditionally, Teochew cuisine embraces lighter cooking techniques, such as steaming, poaching, and quick stir-fries. Seasonings are used sparingly, primarily to enhance the natural freshness of ingredients during food preparation. Thus, Teochew dishes are usually prepared with light and clean soup bases instead of robust and complex flavours. Teochew cuisine is considered one of the healthiest Chinese cuisines due to its cooking philosophies and eating habits. This style of cooking emphasises clean eating for many centuries, long before it became trendy.

The Birth of Myrita2

Hence, *Myrita2* was born. It is a space to pause, ponder, and prosper about how to improve one's health. *Myrita2* is a collection of sixteen recipes, using mostly fruits and vegetables, that I use at home to nourish my family and loved ones. These fruits and vegetables are natural remedies that are commonly available at most of our grocery stores. I am inspired by rainbow diet and clean eating.

In this booklet, I aim to share all-natural remedies from Eastern and Western traditions which are accessible to most people everywhere. None of the recipes claims to be a cure-all to good health. However, each entry aims to raise awareness of the myriad of wholesome goodness that Mother Nature has blessed earthlings with. On top of carbohydrates, proteins, and fats, there are over 4,000 types of phytochemicals or phytonutrients found in fruits and vegetables, each phytochemical offers a host of health-promoting functions and immunity boosters. We can find many natural remedies within easy access without having to defer to ultraprocessed foods and chemical compounds.

In light of the COVID-19 pandemic that is sweeping across the world during the writing of this booklet, this is particularly handy. The human race is confronted by an unparalleled wave of uncertainty and gloom. In the absence of scientifically proven therapeutics and vaccines available at the time of writing, leading health experts recommend frequent washing hands with soap and wearing face masks when in public so as to combat COVID-19. Additionally, we are advised to maintain regular exercise and boost our immunity system by eating more fresh fruits and vegetables.

All recipes in *Myrita2* serve four persons. You are encouraged to modify the quantity and ingredients according to your personal preferences and local market availability. While you develop your cooking skills and confidence, you may occasionally buy the wrong ingredients, burn some pots and pans, or scald your fingers. Just like I did. Whenever possible, I include suggestions in the recipes to widen the cooking options, which vary according to local environment and individual situations. As more green activists and eco-warriors steer towards plant-based diets, no meat is used in these recipes. Dairy products and eggs are required sparingly. For readers with strict dietary restrictions, the dairy products and eggs can be easily substituted. No animal is harmed in the production of *Myrita2*. I have tested most recipes in different locations that I have lived in - Singapore, Perth (Australia), Kuala Lumpur (Malaysia), Boulogne-Billancourt (France), and Shanghai (China).

In the spirit of growth and learning, *Myrita2* nudges her readers to experiment and explore with different local seasonal produce. The kitchen is a fun and fantastic laboratory. Different combinations of ingredients yield different taste profiles. However, do note that certain ingredients may clash when eaten together. For example, tofu and spinach are not to be consumed concurrently. Do your research before you try new combinations. In the reference pages, a list of credible resources is curated for you to expand your culinary repertoire.

To enhance the atmosphere during mealtimes, consider dressing up the dining table, playing soothing music, keeping all mobile devices away, and just eat. These gestures elevate your mood and allow you to mindfully practise self-care.

Begin your healthy lifestyle by examining your daily activities and consumption habits. Purchase fresh produce whenever possible. Wash raw food thoroughly before preparation and consumption. Good hygiene prevails in the cooking environment to maintain good health.

The human body is a complex organism made up of cardiovascular, central nervous systems, endocrinal, gastrointestinal, lymphatic, immune, skeletal, muscular and vascular systems, reproductive organs, respiratory system, urinary system, cells, skin, and specialised tissues. Health comprises of sports, exercise, stress management, healthcare, friends, diet, hygiene, environment, lifestyle and nutrition. The emphasis of *Myrita2* is on diet, nutrition, with additional tips on other aspects of health. A list of additional resources is curated for you to study further.

Every human body has a different constitution. If you pay close attention, you can monitor and observe any noticeable physical changes. Adapt accordingly. A food journal is added to this booklet to aid you in keeping track of your food intake.

As the sage Plato once extolled, "Knowledge is the food of the soul." This booklet is a handy guide with tips and toolkits on food hygiene, physical activity and hydration. These are carefully curated to help the self-directed earthling become a healthier version of yourself.

Myrita2 may be adapted to your health food shops, bubble tea stall, café, workplace cafeteria, bespoke restaurant, or wellness centre. You may contact me for a chat over a glass of natural remedy at myritabook@gmail.com.

Every meal is an opportunity for you to nourish your body. May we all be well and happy and safe.

Bon appétit.

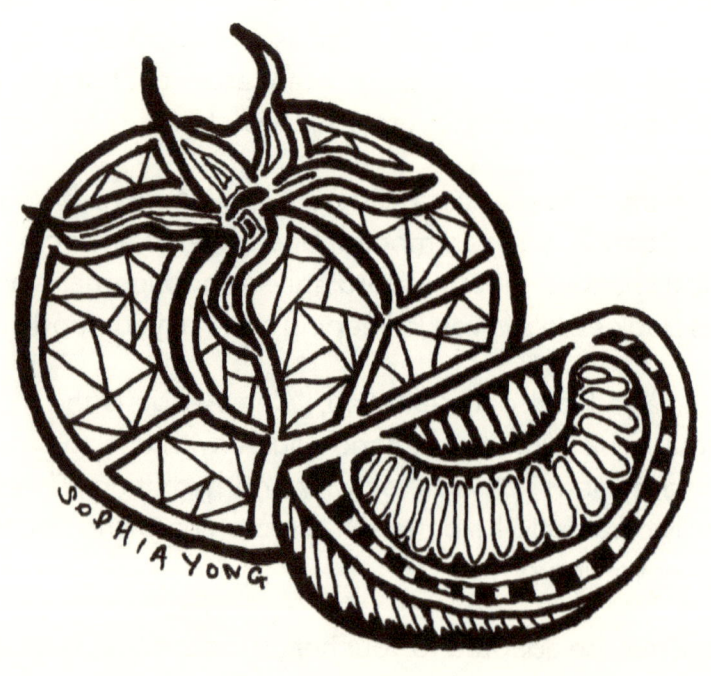

Part A

Your Commitment

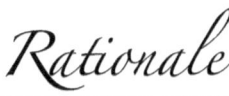

Rationale

Why are your health and fitness goals important? Explain.

1.

2.

3.

4.

5.

My Learning Contract

I, _____ [name],

am ready to become a slightly healthier version of myself. I have made a firm decision to reach

_____

_____

_____

[specify health/fitness goals, timeline].

Signature:
Date:

Part B

Sixteen All-Natural Recipes and Immunity Boosters

Zealous Passion Fruit Coconut Water

Passion fruit is a yellow or purple fruit that grows in warm tropical climate. As it ripens, the skin wrinkles to indicate a higher level of natural sweetness. When a passion fruit is cut open, the soft pulp holds a lot of edible seeds. It contains high levels of vitamin A, which is important for skin, vision, and the immune system; and vitamin C, which is an important antioxidant. It also has traces of potassium, magnesium, iron, and calcium. With a low glycaemic index, passion fruit contains plenty of dietary fibre that is crucial for regulating digestive system and keeping the gut happy.

    3 to 5 ripe passion fruits
    1 fresh coconut with pulp
    500 ml drinking water
    ice cubes (optional)

Cut the passion fruits into halves. Remove the fleshy pulp and seeds and put into a mixing bowl.
Pour coconut water into the mixing bowl.
Scrape the pulp of the coconut from the inside, cut the coconut pulp into small pieces, and add to the mixing bowl.
Ladle all ingredients in the mixing bowl. Stir well.
Add water and/or ice cubes, if required.
Serve in tall glasses with long spoons and/or reusable straws.
Gaze into the fruity concoction and sip calmly.

- ༀ If fresh coconut is unavailable, packaged coconut water may be used.
- ༀ Freshly brewed green tea is an excellent variation to water.
- ༀ Freshly squeezed orange juice is another awesome alternative.
- ༀ Bubbly spring water is a luxurious liquid for special occasions.
- ༀ You may blend the juice for a smoother texture.

Zesty Triple Citrus Juice

Oranges, clementines/tangerines, mandarin oranges, grapefruits, lemons, limes, and pomelos belong to the citrus family. Generally, they are rich in vitamins A and C and packed with antioxidants. These can help combat the formation of free radicals, which health experts believe give rise to cancer. The combination of fibre, choline, lycopene, potassium, and vitamin C, found in citrus fruits, could all contribute to heart health, regulate blood pressure, and prevent stroke. Citrus fruits have high levels of water and fibre. Both water and fibre aid to prevent constipation and promote regularity for a healthy digestive system.

This zesty concoction is a delightful beverage. For optimal fibre consumption and reduction of food waste, my preference is to consume both juice and pulp.

> 1 to 2 oranges, remove skin and cut into quarters
> 1 to 2 grapefruits, remove skin and cut into quarters
> 1 lemon, remove skin and cut into quarters (optional, 2 to 3 limes)
> 2 glasses of water (optional)
> ice cubes (optional)

Put all the citrus fruits into an electric blender. Blend until smooth.
Add 2 glasses of water and/or ice cubes, if preferred.
Serve in long glasses with long spoons and/or reusable straws. Observe your zesty refreshment and recharge with this uplifting experience.

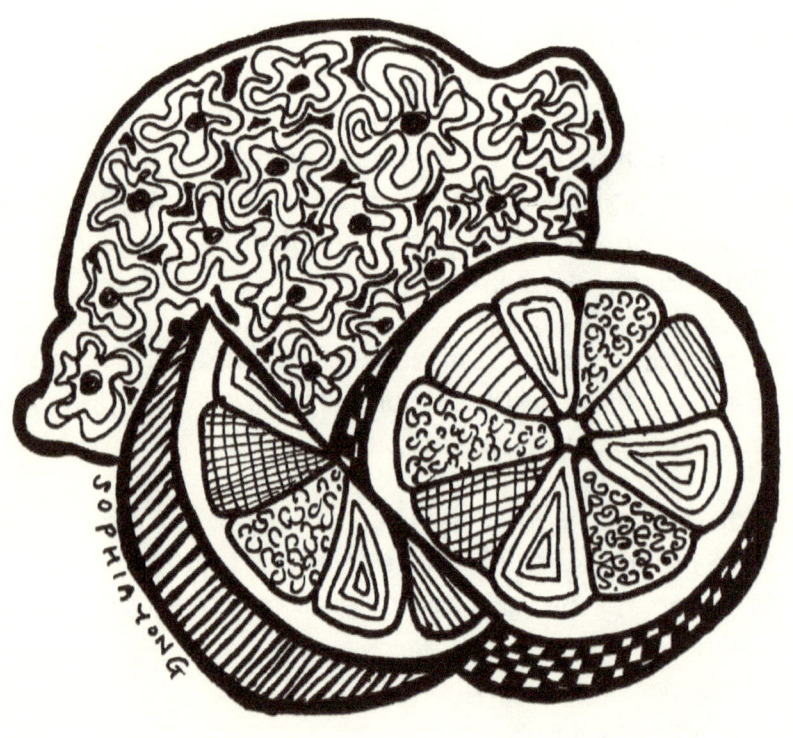

Cool Cucumber Mint Water

Cucumber is classified as a fruit but eaten like a vegetable. With 90 per cent water content, it is highly hydrating. Cucumber contains calcium, magnesium, potassium, phosphorous, and vitamins A and K. Cucumber water has many benefits, including weight loss, hydration, blood pressure management, and skin health. This recipe is affordable, easy to make, and an excellent substitute for sugary carbonated drinks.

> 2 to 3 cucumbers, peeled and cut into 3 cm sticks
> 4 to 5 small limes, cut half and the juice squeezed out (optional)
> handful of fresh mint leaves
> 500 ml water
> ice cubes (optional)

Mix all ingredients into a jug. Press gently to extract the natural juice.
Serve in long glasses.
Observe the floating fibres and cool down.

Minty Watermelon Cooler

Watermelon has 92 per cent water content and is one of the most hydrating fruits. With a low glycaemic index and low carbohydrates, watermelon is a low-calorie summer snack. Lycopene is a phytonutrient that contributes to the natural cherry-red colour of watermelon. In some medical studies, lycopene is found to curb diabetes and some cancer. Choline is another antioxidant that is found in watermelon. Choline contributes to bodily movements and brain functions. Easily digestible, watermelon contains calcium, folate, magnesium, phosphorous, potassium, and vitamins A, B, and C.

> half a large red watermelon
> 20 to 30 fresh mint leaves
> 500 ml water
> ice cubes (optional)

Cut the watermelon into chunks. Crush with a fork.
Alternatively, you may use an electric blender or food processor to reduce the flesh.
Add water and stir well.
Serve in tall drinking glasses. Top off with fresh mint leaves and ice cubes.
Sit still and slow down your breathing.
Savour the fruity refreshment.

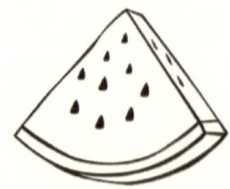

Green Goddess Juice

Kiwi fruit originates from China, brought to New Zealand, and subsequently commercialised. A nutrient powerhouse, kiwi fruit is reputed as a health food due to its high content of vitamin C. Additionally, kiwi fruit contains calcium, folate, lutein, phosphorous, potassium, and vitamins E and K. These nutrients help reduce blood pressure, boost wound healing, help improve bowel health, and maintain glowing skin.

   2 celery sticks, cut into large pieces
   2 green apples, cut into large pieces
   4 green kiwi fruits, peeled and cut into quarters
   2 cucumbers, peeled and cut into large pieces
   ice cubes (optional)

Place all the ingredients into an electric blender. Blend until all the ingredients are smooth.
Serve in tall drinking glasses. Garnish each glass with celery sticks and add ice cubes.
Lengthen your breathing and sip the green juice calmly.

   ꙮ For variations, add green vegetables, such as kale and spinach, to your Green Goddess Juice.

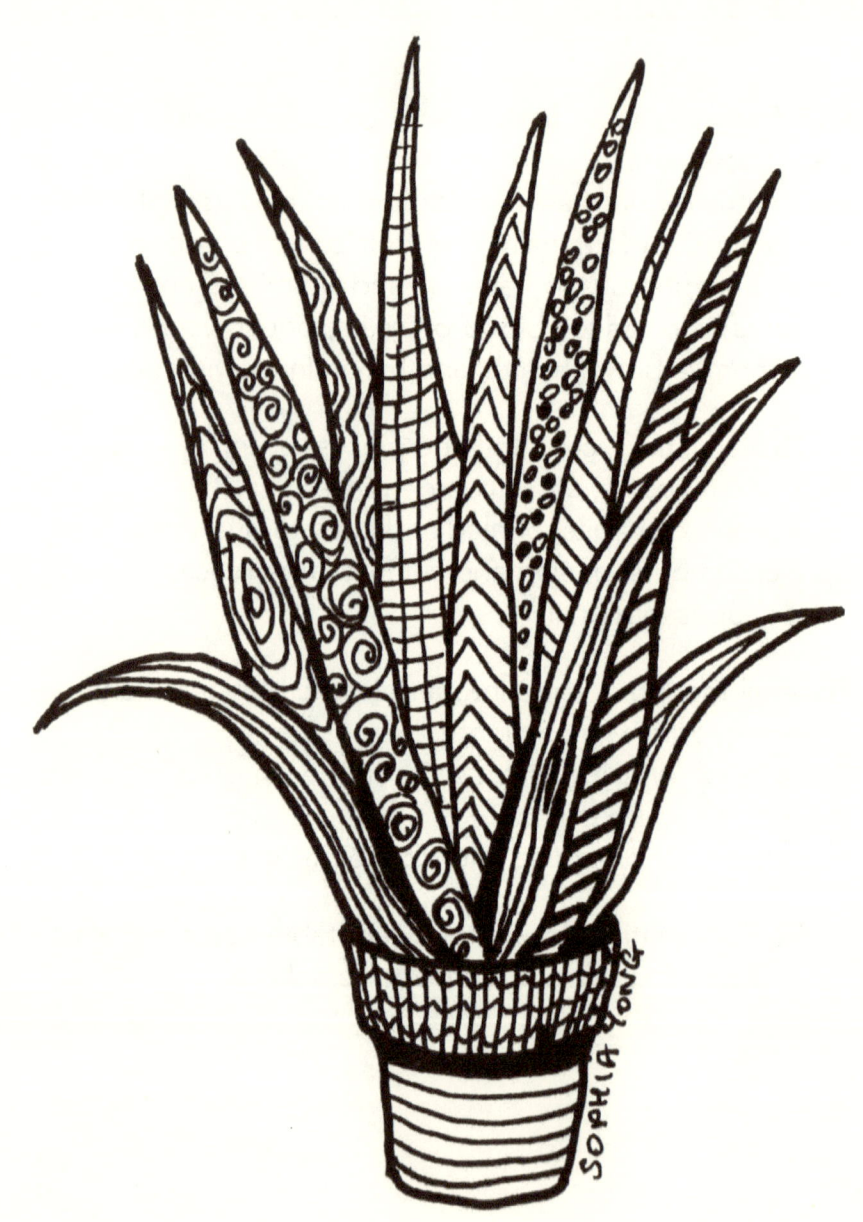

Awesome Aloe Vera Lemonade

Aloe vera is a succulent plant and evergreen perennial. It grows in warm tropical climate and is extensively used in the beauty and cosmetics industry. In some cultures, it is a popular medicinal plant that is known to heal wounds and skin injuries due to its antibacterial, antiviral, and antiseptic properties. A mild laxative, aloe vera is used by Chinese herbalists to smoothen intestinal and stomach function by neutralising toxins and killing parasites.

> 2 to 3 medium-sized aloe vera leaves, cut and scrape translucent gel from the leaves
> 2 to 3 lemons, squeeze out the juice
> 2 to 3 teaspoons of natural honey, dissolve in a half a glass of water (optional)
> 800 ml water
> ice cubes (optional)

Put the gel of aloe vera into a small saucepan. Add half-cup water. Bring to a gentle boil and simmer for about 5 mins.
Combine the cooked aloe vera, lemon juice, and water/ice into a jug.
Mix and serve in long glasses.
Breathe gently and sip the concoction gradually.

> ༄ Limes may be used as an alternative of, or in combination with, lemon.
> ༄ There are remnants of gel on the inside of aloe vera leaves after scraping. Rub the remnant gel on your skin to improve complexion. Discard after use or add to the compost bin.

Cherish Cinnamon Apple Tea

Cinnamon derives from the inner bark of a tropical evergreen tree. The bark is peeled and laid in the sun to dry, where it curls up into rolls known as cinnamon sticks. It also comes in powdered form. Chinese herbalists use cinnamon for its antiviral, antibacterial, and antifungal properties. This aromatic spice also contains large amounts of polyphenol antioxidants, which have anti-inflammatory effects. Its prebiotic properties promote the growth of beneficial bacteria, which suppress the growth of pathogenic bacteria. Thus, add cinnamon regularly in your diet to help improve gut health.

>   half a red apple, sliced thinly
>   1 cinnamon stick
>   1 L of boiling water
>   2 to 3 tsp of English breakfast tea leaves
>   3 to 4 tsp of brown or palm sugar (optional)
>   ice cubes (optional)

In a small saucepan, pour half the boiling water. Add the apple slices.
Simmer the apple slices with cinnamon and brown sugar, until the apple slices soften.

In a teapot, pour the other half of the boiling water to the tea leaves. Steep for approximately 5 mins.
In a larger jug, combine both sets of liquid and stir thoroughly. Serve in teacups.

Inhale the aromatic tea and drink mindfully.

- ℞ For a chilled drink, cool down the beverage and add ice cubes. Refrigerate for two hours before serving.
- ℞ Honey may be used instead of sugar.

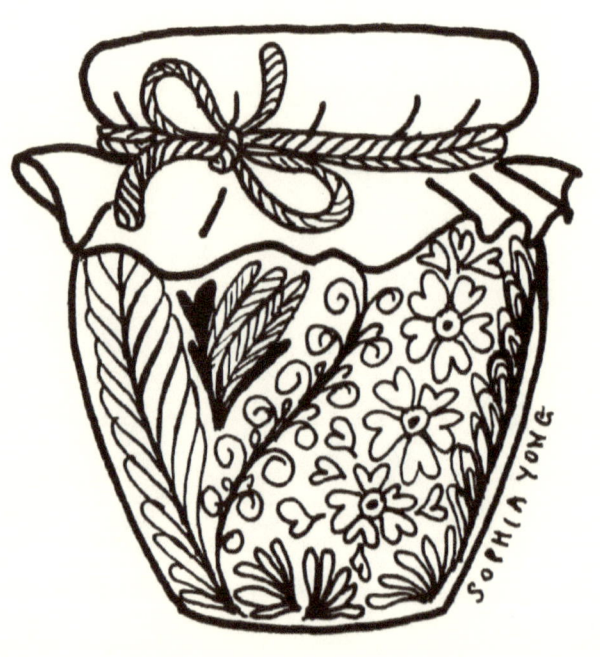

Himalayan Honey Ginger Tea

Ginger is an underground root with a spicy fragrance. A popular ingredient used in many Asian cooking, it is usually sliced, chopped, pounded, or grounded. Sometimes, the juice is extracted and used. Mature ginger has richer scent and taste. Used for thousands of years in traditional Ayurvedic, Arabic, and Chinese medicines, ginger is reputed for treating ailments such as indigestion, flatulence, nausea, joint pain, or motion sickness.

    5 to 8 cm of old ginger, grated
    2 to 3 lemons, quartered and the juice squeezed out
    3 to 5 tsp honey
    1 L boiling water

Combine all ingredients in a teapot.
Pour boiling water into tea teapot and steep for 10 to 20 mins.
Sieve, pour the liquid into teacups. Garnish with thin lemon slices.
You are recommended to consume this in the morning to wake the body.
Inhale the rich aroma, gaze into the golden liquid, and sip the nourishing hot tea.

Vivid Vegetables Soup Stock

Carrot is a root vegetable and raved as the ultimate health food. While the sweet, crunchy, and aromatic orange variety is popular, there are also purple, red, yellow, and white carrots. Carrot is rich in antioxidants that may help to prevent age-related macular degeneration, which is a type of vision loss. Carrot provides beta-carotene, folate, iron, lutein, phosphorous, potassium, zeaxanthin, and vitamins A, C, E, and K.

1 to 2 carrots, cut into chunks
2 to 3 sticks celery, cut into 3 cm sticks
1 to 2 white onions, cut into large cubes
1 to 2 sticks leek, cut into large cubes
2 L boiling water

Fine sea salt
20 to 30 peppercorns, cracked

Put all the cut vegetables into a large saucepan. Add boiling water.
Bring to boil, then turn to low heat. Simmer for 2 to 3 hours.
Add salt and pepper to taste
Cool down the soup stock, strain, and portion into 3 to 5 medium-sized containers.
Refrigerate for up to 3 days, if you wish to use later.

- If you use a slow cooker, stew the soup stock for 3 to 4 hours.
- To minimise food waste, vegetable scraps, such as cauliflower/broccoli stalks, may be added to the

ingredients. These vegetable scraps also enhance the flavour of the soup stock while adding nutritional value.

- If you are using the soup stock for later, you can freeze for up to 2 months for subsequent use.
- Defrost and bring to boil before use for soups.

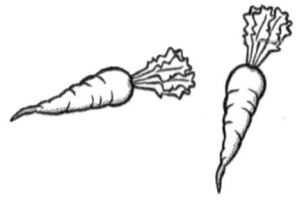

Plush Pumpkin Stew

Pumpkin is a roundish orange vegetable. A member of the squash family, pumpkin is a highly nutritious food that is rich in fibre and low in calorie. Research studies indicate that pumpkin may regulate blood pressure, reduce the risk of cancer, protect against age-related eye diseases, and prevent and control diabetes. Pumpkin provides folate, iron, magnesium, phosphorous, zinc, copper, and vitamins A, C, and E.

1.5 kg butternut pumpkin (also called squash), peeled and cut into large chunks
3 large white onions, peeled and cut into large chunks
1.5 L vegetable soup stock
2 cloves of garlic, peeled and crushed
2 to 3 bay leaves

30 g unsalted butter
1 tsp paprika
salt and pepper to taste

Garnish (optional items)
dried Italian herbs
half-cup thick cream

In a large saucepan, melt the butter and cook the onion until it starts to brown. Add the pumpkin and cook until it starts to brown.
Add the soup stock and bring it to a boil.
Add bay leaves, salt, and pepper. Simmer for about an hour.
Turn off the heat and cool off the soup. Remove the bay leaves.
With an electric blender, blend the cooled soup.

Return the blended soup to the saucepan. Heat up the soup.
Add the paprika.
Serve the soup, with the garnish you prefer.
Slowly savour your hearty autumn soup.

- ℞ Chicken stock is an option for those who prefer a meaty enhancement.
- ℞ This recipe may be stewed for 3 to 4 hours in a slow cooker.
- ℞ Thick cream may be added to the soup upon serving, if you prefer.

Delicate Egg Flower Soup

In north and central China, the eggy flower soup is a popular dish that is quick and easy to prepare. It usually accompanies an evening meal with other dishes. In this recipe, I add seaweed, tofu, and tomato to enhance the nutritional contents of this light broth. In Chinese, it is known as 蛋花汤 (pronounced: *dàn huā tāng*).

> 800 ml vegetable soup stock
> 1 to 2 eggs, beaten
> 2 ripe large tomatoes, cut into cubes
> 1 pack soft or silken tofu, cut into large cubes (optional)
>
> soya sauce
> sesame oil
> white pepper powder
>
> Garnish (optional items)
> 1 to 2 sheets of seaweed or nori, shredded
> a sprig of spring onion and/or Chinese parsley, chopped finely
> 2 to 3 tsp fried shallots

In a saucepan, bring soup stock to a boil.
Add tomatoes; bring to a boil.
Add soft tofu.
Gently drip the beaten egg in a narrow stream along the prongs of a fork into the soup stock, trailing it over the surface. Wait 15 seconds for the egg to start to set. Gently stir 2 to 3 times. Let the soup simmer.

When the egg is cooked, it spreads out in the soup like a blooming flower, hence the name bestowed on this simple dish.

Drizzle your preferred amount of seasoning.

Serve in a family soup bowl.

Garnish with seaweed, fried shallots, and chopped spring onion/Chinese parsley.

Slowly savour this delicate and digestible broth.

℞ Dried scallops or dried abalone may be added to the soup to enhance its flavour.

℞ For a more robust flavour, chicken or pork bone soup stock may be used instead of vegetable soup stock.

Wondrous Winter Melon Soup

Goji berries, or Chinese wolfberries, are red seeds from a plant in Northeast Asia and Inner Mongolia. Chinese physicians have used goji berries for centuries to help improve vision and renal function. Goji berries contain several phytochemicals, including (1) polysaccharides, which is a vital source of dietary fibre that may improve immune function and increase total antioxidant activity in the body; (2) beta-carotene, which is essential for eye health, bone health, skin health, and cell development; and (3) zeaxanthin, which supports the immune system. Potentially, these phytochemicals may slow down macular degeneration of the eye retina.

800 ml vegetable soup stock
400 g winter melon, peeled, pith removed and cut into chunks
1 large carrot, peel and cut into chunks
4 shiitake mushrooms, cut into quarters
3 tsp goji berries, rinsed and drained

soya sauce
sesame oil
white pepper powder

Garnish (optional items)
1 to 2 sheets of seaweed or nori, shredded
1 to 2 sprigs of spring onion or Chinese parsley, chopped finely
2 to 3 tsp of fried shallots

In a medium saucepan, bring soup stock to a boil.

Place the mushrooms in the soup and simmer for 5 mins.
Add winter melon, carrot, and goji berries. Bring to a boil and
simmer for 20 to 30 mins.

Add your preferred amount of seasoning.
Serve in individual soup bowls.
Garnish with seaweed, fried shallots, and chopped spring
onion/Chinese parsley.
Sit still. Savour this mild broth.

- Dried scallops or dried abalone may be added to the soup to enhance its flavour.
- For a more robust flavour, chicken or pork bone soup stock may be used instead of vegetable soup stock.

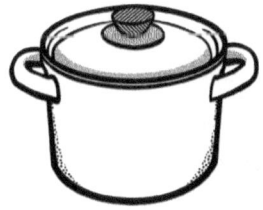

Rainbow Salad with Asian Dressing

This vibrant salad is inspired by the wide variety of colourful natural foods available at the fresh food section of many urban grocery stores. The Asian-style dressing hints of new flavours and another gastronomic wonderland.

Alfalfa belongs to the sprouts family. Sprouts are immature plants with little shoots that start to grow when a seed germinates. The curly vegetable has a mild, grassy flavour. This microgreen is a rich source of vitamin K and a decent source of copper, folate, iron, magnesium, phosphorous, zinc, and vitamin C. Due to the significant level of vitamin K, alfalfa is highly recommended for building bones. Research studies demonstrate that alfalfa may reduce cholesterol while reducing inflammation. Alfalfa contains protein and is low in calorie count.

1 cup raw chickpeas
10 baby or cherry tomatoes, halved
10 baby carrots, halved
1 capsicum, sliced thinly
2 pieces firm tofu, diced and pan-fried
1 head of lettuce of your choice, shredded thickly

Asian-style dressing:
2 tsp extra virgin olive oil
1 tsp soy sauce
1 tsp sesame oil
2 tsp rice vinegar
2 tsp fried shallot and/or garlic

Garnish (optional items)
handful of alfalfa
1 to 2 tsp pumpkin and/or sunflower seeds
1 to 2 tsp roasted white sesame

Soak the raw chickpeas overnight in water. Drain and cook in boiling water for about 45 mins, or until softened. When cooked, drain off the water, and cool down the chickpeas.

Combine the vegetable ingredients in a salad mixing bowl.
To make the dressing, combine the ingredients of the dressing in a separate mixing bowl. Stir and mix well.
Pour the dressing into the large mixing bowl. Toss well.
Serve in individual salad bowls. Top off each serving with the garnish you prefer.
Chew each mouthful of your salad deliberately.
Bon appétit.

- Lemon juice may replace rice vinegar for the dressing. Extract freshly squeezed lemon juice from 1 fruit for this purpose.
- For non-vegetarians, boiled quail eggs is an interesting addition of protein.
- Avocado is another delicious and nourishing addition to this vibrant dish.

Vibrant Steamed Vegetables

Walnut is the edible seed of a drupe. It is popularly thought that walnut is a brain food simply because its shape resembles the human brain. Walnut contains plenty of polyunsaturated fatty acids, which are healthier than saturated fats. Additionally, walnuts have alpha-linolenic and linoleic acids, which may have anti-inflammatory effects that keep blood vessels healthy. Walnut is also rich in vitamin E and iron. A handful of raw or roasted walnuts a day is recommended for a balanced diet.

1 large broccoli, or cauliflower, cut into 3 cm florets
1 carrot, peeled and cut into 3 cm sticks
10 young corns, cut into 3 cm pieces
10 baby asparagus, cut into 3 cm sticks
10 Brussels sprouts, cut into halves

Asian-style dressing:
2 tsp extra virgin olive oil
1 tsp sesame oil
2 tsp soy sauce
2 tsp rice vinegar
2 tsp of fried shallot and/or garlic

Garnish (optional items)
handful of alfalfa
1 to 2 tsp of chia seeds
1 to 2 tsp of roasted black sesame seeds
handful of raw walnuts, chopped finely

In a large saucepan or rice cooker, set up the equipment for steaming. When the water is at boiling temperature, the steaming equipment is ready.

Place all the vegetables in the steaming basket. Steam for 4 to 6 mins.

In a small mixing bowl, mix all the ingredients of the dressing. Remove vegetables from the steamer, then serve in salad bowls. Add dressing and garnish.

Observe your vibrant meal and give thanks to the nourishment from Mother Nature.

Bon appétit.

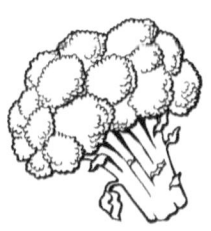

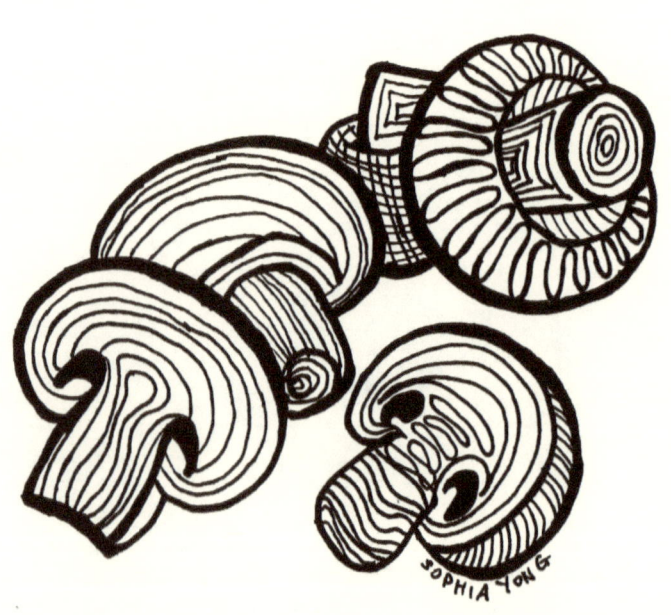

Marvellous Mushroom Omelette

Over 2,000 edible mushrooms are found in nature, but only a handful are available in consumer markets. Edible mushrooms include button (or white), brown, enoki, oyster, portobello, shiitake, truffle, and wood ear (or black fungus). Though they contain over 90 per cent water, mushrooms have protein; vitamins B2, B3, and B5; plus calcium, copper, iron, phosphorous, potassium, and selenium. The choline in mushrooms can help with muscle movement and keeping a healthy brain. Historical records have demonstrated that this all-natural multivitamin is used in some types of traditional medicine.

You should only eat mushrooms from a reliable source as some types are toxic.

3 to 4 eggs medium-sized eggs
1 large onion, sliced finely
4 to 5 shiitake or button mushrooms, sliced finely
1 capsicum, colour of your choice, cut into thin strips
10 to 20 leaves of fresh basil leaves
handful of alfalfa for garnish and added nutrition (optional)
slices of cheddar/mozzarella cheese (optional)

pinch of sea salt
ground white pepper
2 tbs cooking oil
dried Italian herbs (optional)

In a frying pan, heat up the oil. Fry the onion till it starts to brown a little.

Sauté mushroom until it softens.
Add capsicum and basil till they start to soften. Set the half-cooked ingredients aside.
Add dried Italian herbs.

Add more oil to the frying pan if necessary.
Pour a quarter portion of beaten egg into the frying pan. Put on low fire until it starts to firm up.
Add one-quarter of the cooked vegetables. Fold the omelette in half. Cook to the preferred level of firmness. Repeat this step multiple times.

Serve on dinner plates.
Nourish yourself with every morsel of omelette.

    ☈ If you like a cheesy omelette, add slices of cheddar or mozzarella cheese when the egg is half-cooked. Fold the omelette and wait until it is almost firm.

Lala's Beetroot Salad with Tropical Twist

Beetroot is a fibrous root vegetable. It eases digestion, which is essential for a healthy gut. It also contains folate, iron, magnesium, phosphorous, and vitamins A and C. Beetroot provides alpha-lipoic acid, which is an antioxidant that may lower glucose levels and increase insulin sensitivity. Beetroot provides a wide range of possible health benefits, such as reduced blood pressure, improved digestion, and lowered risk for diabetes.

1 beetroot
25 g roasted cashew nuts, chopped finely
2 cm fresh ginger, peeled and grated
3 tbs coconut cream
1 tbs lemon juice
0.5 tsp cumin powder
0.5 tsp salt

Wash beetroot, and cook it in lightly salted water for 45 mins. Peel the cooked beetroot and let it cool down.
Grate the cooked beetroot, then squeeze out the beetroot juice. Set aside the juice for other uses.
Mix all the ingredients (grated beetroot, cashews, ginger, coconut cream, lemon juice, cumin, and salt) together.
Chill in the fridge for 1 to 2 hours. Serve the salad when the rest of the meal is ready.
When eating, just eat.

છ Retain the beetroot juice. It may be used as natural colouring for dips, hummus, soups, deserts, cakes, etc.

♥ This recipe is contributed by Lala Olga Wagner.

Part C

More Useful Health Tips

Healthy-Eating Shopping List

Rainbow Diet

The secret to healthy bones, sharp memory, youthful skin, and disease prevention can be found in your refrigerator. The more colourful your diet is, the more antioxidants you get. Antioxidants reduce overall cellular damage and prevent the hardening of the arteries that can lead to heart disease, stroke, and even memory loss. Every hue - green, yellow, orange, red, purple, and even white - signifies a different class of nutrients, each of which offers a unique benefit. Hence, the concept of rainbow diet comes about.

There are over 4,000 types of phytochemicals or phytonutrients in plants and vegetables. Essentially, phytochemicals are chemicals produced by plants, often with specific nutritional value. These phytochemicals in plants offer the possibility of improving your health in various ways, such as lowering cholesterol, enhancing immune system, and having antiseptic, antibacterial, antifungal, antimicrobial, antioxidant, anti-inflammatory, and anticancer properties.

→ Aim for "five a day" portions of fruits and vegetables. An average person needs to consume 400 g of fruits and vegetables a day, that is, five portions of 80 g.

→ Target to eat two fruits each day. Buy at least three different types of fruits each week.

→ Every week, buy at least three different fresh vegetables, of different colours.

→ For an age-defying eating plan, mix and match these colours to ensure variety at your meals. Research indicates that antioxidants are better off working together like a team, each boosting the other's effects.

| Green | * High content of chlorophyll, which gives it the colour.
* Rich in vitamin K, lutein, folate, iron, and zeaxanthin.
* May curb the growth of certain cancer cells.
* Slow cognitive decline.
* Aid eye health.
* Enhance immune system response. | arugula (rocket)
asparagus
avocado
basil
pak choi
broccoli
Brussels sprouts
celery
choi sum (cai-xin)
cucumber
green beans
green capsicum (bell pepper)
green grapes
kale
kiwi
leek
lettuce
lime
microgreens (e.g. alfalfa)
okra (lady's fingers)
peas
pears
spinach
watercress
zucchini |

Yellow/ Orange	* Rich in beta-carotene, which gives rise to vitamin A. * Essential for vision, growth, and development.	apricots carrots corn ginger mango melons peaches pineapple pumpkin (squash) rock melon (cantaloupe) sweet potatoes tangerines (clementines) yellow capsicum (bell pepper)
Blue/ Purple	* Rich in antioxidants. * High in nitrates. * Helps to reduce blood pressure.	aubergine (eggplant) blackberries blueberries dates figs purple grapes prunes raisins

Red	* Rich in carotenoid and lycopene. * Helps to reduce risk of certain cancers, such as prostate cancer.	beetroot cherries cranberries pink grapefruit raspberries red apples red capsicum (bell pepper) red grapes strawberries tomatoes watermelons
White	* Contains vitamins B1 and B2, which help the body get energy from food and form red blood cells. * Important for a healthy brain. * Essential for metabolism, healthy skin, eyes, and nervous system.	banana cabbage cauliflower chickpeas garlic mushrooms onion parsnip potatoes

Grains

Whole grains are unrefined grains that have not had their bran and germ removed by milling. Therefore, most of the nutrients remain intact. They provide a variety of healthy nutrients and are naturally low in fat. Whole grains are better sources of fibre and other important nutrients, such as selenium, potassium, and magnesium. There is a variety of whole grains, and it is best to avoid refined and enriched grains.

Examples of whole grains include the following

- ☐ barley
- ☐ brown/black/red rice
- ☐ buckwheat
- ☐ millet
- ☐ oatmeal
- ☐ quinoa
- ☐ popcorn
- ☐ rye
- ☐ wholewheat bread, pasta, or crackers
- ☐ wild rice

Generally, whole grains are a good source of calories, carbohydrates, fibre, proteins, B vitamins, and phytochemicals. Most grains contain about 70 to 75 per cent carbohydrate, 10 to 15 per cent protein, 4 to 18 per cent fibre, and 1 to 5 per cent fat. However, the different grains vary in their specific nutritional content. Investigate and consume thoughtfully.

Eat a variety of whole grains to obtain more health-promoting nutrients. It also makes your meals and snacks more interesting. For people with gastro-intestinal issues, you are recommended to consult with medical professionals to ascertain if consuming whole grains is suitable.

Tips to include more whole grains to your meals and snacks:

- ♥ Savour breakfasts that include wholegrain cereals, such as bran flakes, shredded wheat, or oatmeal.
- ♥ Substitute the plain with wholewheat toast or wholegrain bagels. Substitute pastries with low-fat bran muffins.
- ♥ Make sandwiches using wholegrain breads or rolls. Replace white-flour tortillas with wholewheat versions.
- ♥ Replace white rice with brown rice, wild rice, millet, or quinoa.
- ♥ Include wild rice or barley in soups, stews, casseroles, and salads.
- ♥ Use whole grains, such as cooked brown rice or wholegrain breadcrumbs, to ground meat or poultry for extra body.
- ♥ Add rolled oats or crushed bran cereal in recipes instead of dry breadcrumbs.

Tea

Tea deserves an encyclopaedia. For many centuries, the Chinese people have cultivated, celebrated, and propagated tea. The academic name of the tea tree is *Camellia sinensis* (L) Kuntze. Historically, the Japanese and Korean communities also feature tea culture. Typically, most Asians do not add sugar and milk in the tea.

When the British colonised parts of Asia, the tea plant was brought to various parts of India, Sri Lanka, and Malaysia for cultivation. Today, popular Western tea blends include Ceylon, Darjeeling, Earl Grey, and English breakfast.

There are six categories of Chinese tea: green, black, yellow, dark, white, and oolong. The beneficial ingredients in tea include polyphenols and vitamin C, which help to keep the human body healthy. Thus, there is a traditional Chinese saying that "tea is the medicine of ten thousand ailments."

For traditional Chinese medicine (TCM), it is important to maintain the original flavour and function of each tea so as to provide effective remedies.

Tea connoisseurs are particular about how tea is cultivated, harvested, transported, stored, brewed, served, and drunk. Tea, by itself, is an art and a science; it is worthy of a lifetime study.

Recent scientific research reveals many health benefits of drinking tea, including the following:

- ★ aid digestion and prevent constipation
- ★ alleviate toxicity of heavy metal, anti-radiation
- ★ control bacteria and diminish inflammation

* decrease blood sugar
* diminish smoke toxicity
* dispel the adverse effects of alcohol
* help with anti-ageing
* improve eyesight
* improve mental alertness and cognitive processes
* possess anticancer properties
* prevent tooth decay
* reduce and regulate cholesterol and triglycerides in the blood
* stimulate the central nervous system

Add two to three cups of freshly brewed tea to your weekly healthy lifestyle.

Drink your tea slowly and reverently.
-Thich Nhat Hanh

Tofu

Soya has plenty of proteins and oils, which makes it an extremely useful base for meat substitutes. Fermenting the soya releases its rich cargo of nutrients, and these can then be processed to soya milk and soya products, such as tofu, thousand layers tofu, tempeh, and tofu skin.

Tofu has a long tradition in Asian cuisines, including Japanese, Korean, and Malay/Indonesian variations. Also known as bean curd, tofu comes in soft and firm types, marinated, smoked and fermented. Most tofu is usually bland in flavour but absorbs the flavours of foods with which it is cooked with. A versatile and nutritious food item, tofu can be steamed, fried, or boiled. During your purchase, check shelf life and expiry dates of soya products on the packaging.

Soya is naturally cholesterol-free. It contains polyunsaturated fats, including omega-3. It has all nine essential amino acids you need for healthy muscles and bone. Isoflavones, a plant chemical common in soya foods, seem to mimic the effects of oestrogen. Some research suggests that isoflavones may help strengthen bones in women who have had menopause.

Soya is a good source of potassium. Potassium plays a critical role in regulating bodily system, including moderating your heartbeats, filtering waste from your kidneys to filter waste, and making your nerves work.

Water

Water is the elixir of life. It is one of the Best Six Doctors (see page 66)

A person may survive without food for days or weeks but cannot live more than a few days without water.

Approximately 55 to 60 per cent of the adult body weight is water. Water plays critical functions in the human body by:

* regulating body temperature
* moisturising the skin from inside out and keeping it soft and supple
* being the enabling vehicle for important bodily processes of absorption, transportation of nutrients and oxygen, digestion, and removal of waste products
* smoothening the mucus lining in our digestive and urinary system, respiratory system, and reducing the accumulation of toxins in the human body
* helping to manage weight loss if consumed before a meal as it suppresses the appetite and therefore cuts down the amount of food consumed
* flushing out the excessive waste and toxins, thus preventing unhealthy cellular growth and infections
* assisting to reduce fatigue

Depending on individual body requirements, a person requires 1.6 L to 2.5 L (seven to ten glasses) of water a day. Environmental factors such as temperature and humidity, occupation, medical conditions, and activity level of each person, also determine the appropriate amount of water consumption. Water is also present in other beverages such as gravy, juices, milk, soups, and tea.

Tips for obtaining enough water:

→ When you wake up, drink a glass of lukewarm water on an empty stomach. During your sleep, you become super dehydrated. Also, when you drink prior to breakfast, water activates your brain, kidneys, and gut faster

→ Before leaving the house on a sunny day, drink one to two glasses before you go.

→ Carry a water bottle with you when you are outside.

→ Infuse your drinking water with slices of citrus fruits, herbs, or berries. The flavours enhance the drinking experience and add some essential vitamins and minerals.

→ Place your water bottles in a visible spot so you are reminded to hydrate. If necessary, set automated reminders on your mobile devices or watches to remind you to drink hourly.

Hydrate.

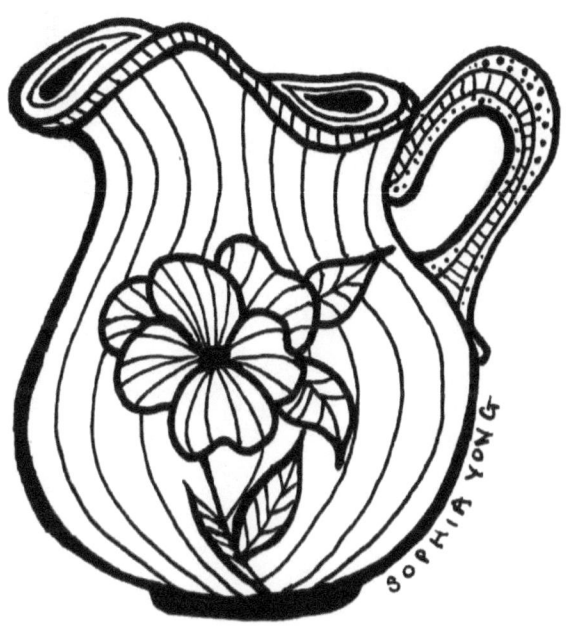

Thirty-One-Day Hydration Challenge

This tool helps you to keep track of your commitment to hydration over a month. Take the thirty-one-day hydration challenge and mark the days you pay attention to how much water you drink a day. Each time you drink a glass of water, reward yourself with a smiley face.

Month		☺	☺	☺	☺	☺	☺	☺	☺
1									
2									
3									
4									
5									
6									
7									
8									
9									
10									
11									
12									
13									
14									
15									
16									
17									
18									
19									
20									
21									
22									
23									
24									
25									
26									
27									
28									
29									
30									
31									

Checklist on Food Hygiene

There are bacteria all around us. Some are good, but others can make us sick or cause food poisoning. *E. coli*, listeria, and salmonella are common culprits. You can shop, store, prepare, and serve food with the best intention for the household. Yet there could be "routine" food handling habits which can breed and spread bacteria. These bacteria can potentially make you and your family very sick. Are you making food hygiene mistakes without realising it?

Thus, it is crucial to maintain cleanliness and hygiene in your kitchen and food storage areas. This is an essential food hygiene checklist for your use.

- ☐ Before food preparation, wash your hands thoroughly with soap and water.
- ☐ Keep raw uncooked meats away from the rest of the groceries. Use separate bags for meat and other items. Throw out the disposable bags that you use to keep the meat. Keep raw and cooked food in separate sections in the kitchen to minimise cross-contamination.
- ☐ After grocery shopping, sort, separate, and store the purchase in your refrigerator and pantry at appropriate temperature. Use good-quality food storage containers so your groceries and ingredients can stay fresh longer; reduce food waste.
- ☐ Wash your reusable shopping bags. Spills and raw meat liquid can carry harmful bacteria.
- ☐ Wash your fruits and vegetables thoroughly to remove unwanted scum. Soak the fresh fruits and vegetables in a basin of tap water, with one to two teaspoons

of coarse salt or baking soda (also known as sodium bicarbonate).

☐ After cooking, consume your meals soon. Do not leave cooked foods and cut fruits and vegetables on the countertops for more than two hours. If you are unable to eat immediately, cool down the cooked dishes, store in good containers, and refrigerate. When you are ready to eat, heat up the refrigerated dishes.

☐ Scrub and disinfect your stove and kitchen countertops with mild soap and water every time you finish cooking. Sweep and mop kitchen floor regularly.

☐ Every five to ten days, wipe the exterior of cabinets, various movable furniture, and equipment to get rid of dust and dirt. Grease builds up and becomes tougher to clean.

☐ Every two to four weeks, clean kitchen equipment such as oven, kettle, toaster, and blender. Maintain these appliances well, and you can prolong their usage and longevity, thus saving money.

☐ Kitchens and dining areas tend to attract house pests such as ants, cockroaches, and lizards. If necessary, use appropriate chemical insecticides sparingly so as to avoid contamination and chemical pollution.

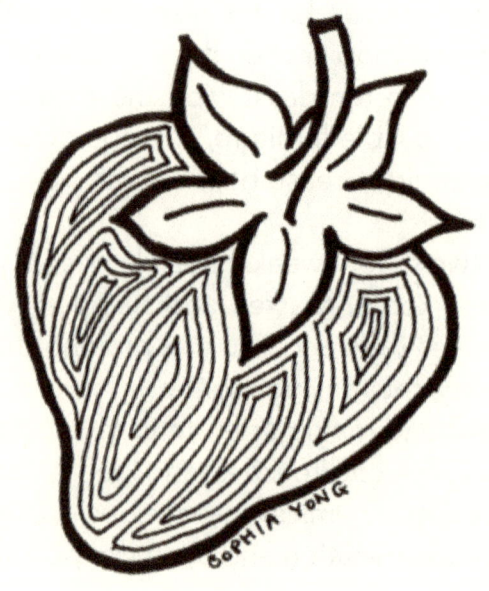

Eat food, not too much, mostly plant.
- Michael Pollan, author of the book Food Rules

Clean Eating

Essentially, clean eating encourages you to consume more whole foods such as fruits, vegetables, lean proteins, whole grains, and healthy fats. At the same time, limit highly processed foods, snacks, sweets, and other packaged foods.

For instance, a wholesome meal containing these nutrients would be a spinach salad with eggs, wild rice, avocado, cashews, and grapes, simply dressed with some olive oil and balsamic vinegar.

Suggestions for clean eating include the following:

→ *Reduce highly processed, packaged foods* with a long list of ingredients, most of which are not natural. Ingredients listed on the food label should mostly be foods that you recognise, such as wholegrain steel-cut oats, dried apple, flaxseed, and cinnamon. Avoid ingredients that you cannot identify or cannot easily pronounce, such as carnauba wax, soy lecithin, and artificial flavouring.

→ *Reduce all foods with added salt, sugar, or fat.*

→ *Avoid foods that are drastically altered compared with their natural form,* such as chicken nuggets versus a fresh chicken breast, apple juice versus a whole apple, or potato chips versus fresh potatoes.

→ There are times when processing can be a positive thing for foods, such as pasteurisation, which makes eggs and dairy products safer for consumption. Also, frozen fruits and vegetables are acceptable because they are minimally processed and can sometimes contain more nutrients than fresh varieties since they are frozen at their peak.

→ *Prepare and eat more foods at home.* Begin with simple meals to ease you get into the habit, such as oatmeal and fresh berries for breakfast or a simple egg fried rice for lunch.

Clean eating is not completely black and white. There is room for adaptation and flexibility, and it does not require avoiding any certain food groups - unless medically necessary.

Clean eating also does not mean consuming raw foods. Cooking, pasteurising, and preserving are fine if excessive seasoning is not used.

Replacing meals with store-bought protein shakes or sugary smoothies and juices is *not* an example of clean eating.

Remove Bad Eating Habits

It is challenging to change your lifestyle and diet. When your pantry and refrigerators are full of ice cream, potato chips, frozen dinners, carbonated drinks, cookies, and candies, it is a mounting task to overcome these temptations.

As you stock up on healthy foods, gradually eliminate the unhealthy ones. Your environments play a crucial role in your food consumption; the mere sight of unhealthy food can stimulate your appetite. While some of these foods may be convenient for your children or other family members, filling your shelves with healthier options will benefit them too. If you are unable to exclude these foods completely from your home, try putting them in places where you will be less tempted. As the saying goes, "Out of sight, out of mind."

Remove or cut down these unhealthy foods from your pantry:

- ✘ bacon and cold cuts that are high in fat or sodium
- ✘ candies, sweets
- ✘ carbonated beverages
- ✘ chicken nuggets
- ✘ chips
- ✘ cookies
- ✘ doughnuts
- ✘ French fries
- ✘ fruit roll-ups
- ✘ full-fat cheese
- ✘ granola bars with added sugars
- ✘ ice cream
- ✘ jam-filled cereal bars

- ✗ muffins
- ✗ popsicles
- ✗ snack cakes
- ✗ soda toaster tarts
- ✗ white bread
- ✗ whole milk crackers (other than wholegrain, low-salt)

Essentially, most packaged foods have high levels of fats, salt, and sugar. Avoid the five food felons - saturated fats, trans fat, refined grains, added syrups, and sugars (anything in the food labels ending with -ose). If you have to, consume these food felons sparingly. Scrutinise food labels and invest in your own health. You will surely reap the benefits in the years to come.

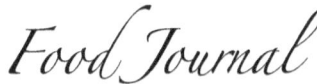

Food Journal

A food journal documents and tracks your intake of food and beverage on a weekly basis. The food journal offers you a space to reflect on your food intake. Over time, you will notice your eating patterns and consumption habits. This is where you can identify red flags and nip the problem in the bud.

Here is a template to record your weekly eating habits. After keeping records over a one-month period, you would notice certain trends and recurring patterns. You may make multiple copies of this template to help you monitor yourself over several weeks or months.

You are what you eat. For people with health issues, identify risks and connections. It is your prerogative to take relevant actions for your state of health.

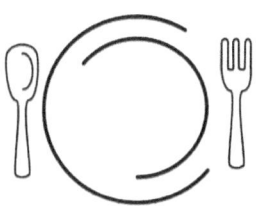

	Monday	Tuesday	Wednesday	Thursday	Friday	Saturday	Sunday	Notes
Breakfast								
Lunch								
Snack								
Dinner								
Eating environment/ companions								
Feelings								
Bodily conditions								

Physical Activity Journal

A lack of physical activity is a significant risk factor for non-communicable diseases such as stroke, diabetes, and cancer. As the urban masses increasingly adopt sedentary lifestyle, less and less physical activity is occurring in many countries. Globally, 23 per cent of adults and 81 per cent of schoolgoing adolescents are not active enough (WHO, 2020).

Regular physical activity helps to maintain a healthy body. When you are physically active, you:

* improve your muscular and respiratory fitness
* improve your bone and functional health
* reduce chances of coronary heart disease, high blood pressure, stroke, diabetes, cancer (including colon and breast cancer), and depression
* reduce the risk of falling, fractures, and broken bones
* are more likely to maintain your weight

Guidelines for level of physical activities:

Age group	Activity level
5 to 17 years old	60 min. a day
18 to 64 years old	150 min. a week
65 years old and above	150 min. a week # Subject to recommendations from physicians and medical professionals

Ageing is inevitable. Our bodily muscles and brain cells shrink as we age. Yet thousands of new cells are created every day. Research shows that regular exercise activates the growth of new cells. Furthermore, regular exercise contributes to better mood and mental wellness.

Ageing gracefully is a personal choice. Suggestions to keep moving include the following:

→ Find a buddy.
→ Get outdoors.
→ Keep it bright.
→ Play funky music.
→ Prepare yourself ahead of time.
→ Sign up for a class for social learning and group synergy.

This physical activity journal documents and tracks your physical movement on a weekly basis. This tool offers you a space to reflect on your level of physical activity. Over time, you will observe your active lifestyle and notice certain trends and recurring patterns. This is where you can identify arising issues and arrest the problems. You will take the necessary actions to align with your health and fitness goals. Duplicate the following template to use it over multiple weeks.

	Monday	Tuesday	Wednesday	Thursday	Friday	Saturday	Sunday	Notes
Morning								
Afternoon								
Evening								
State of mind								
Bodily conditions								

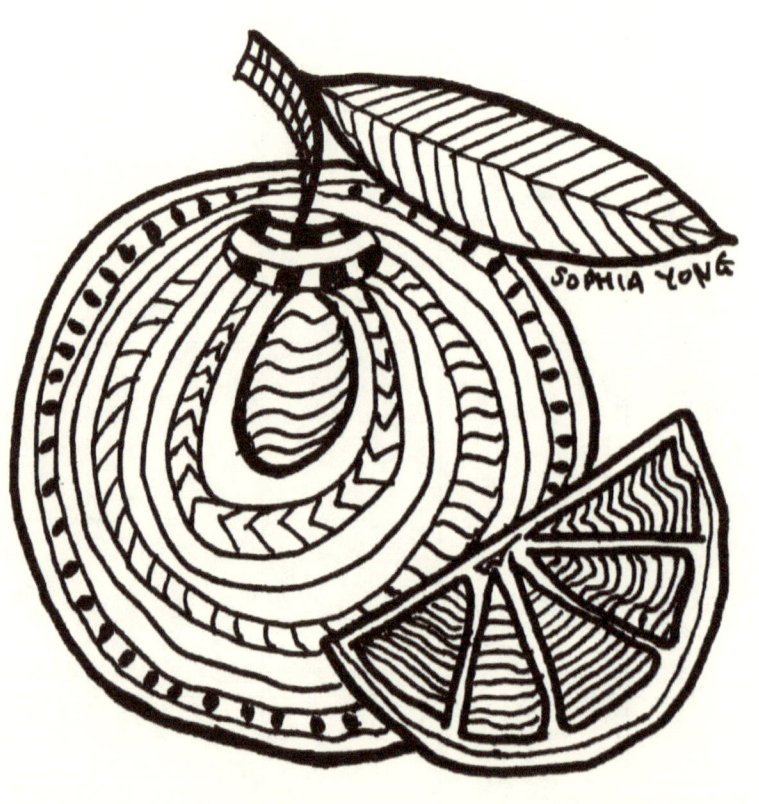

Fitness Bingo

A Japanese proverb goes, "Only staying active will make you want to live a hundred years."

The fitness bingo is a game to help you associate the members of your households, or families, with each particular activity. The more activities each person has, the more physically fit she/he is likely to be.

FITNESS BINGO				
Arm circles	Hops on each foot	Window cleaning	Bicycles	Weightlifting
Sit-up	Dancing	Toe touches	Clean the wardrobes	Skipping
Gardening	Heel raises	Head rotation	Push-up	Reach out to the sky
Squats	Manual car wash	Leg lifts	Walking backwards	Trampoline
Star jumps	Brisk walk	Swimming	Side kicks	Handwash dirty laundry

Rules
Three to eight persons from your household or family are required for this game.
Mingle around. Identify who does any particular activities. Write the person's name in the corresponding activity boxes. The first person who completes one row, or one column, is the winner.

The Best Six Doctors

The best six doctors anywhere, and no one can deny it,
Are sunshine, water, rest, and air, exercise and diet.
These six will gladly you attend, if only you are willing.
Your mind they'll ease.
Your will they'll mend.
And charge you not a shilling.

- Wayne Fields in What the River Knows

I am exceptionally fond of my Best Six Doctors for mental, emotional, and physical well-being. In this space, consider if you are in close contact with these Best Six Doctors to maintain optimal health. Are you committing time to the right doctors?

	How often am I interacting with the right doctors currently?	What do I want to do more of?
Fresh air		
Diet		
Exercise		
Sunshine		
Rest		
Water		

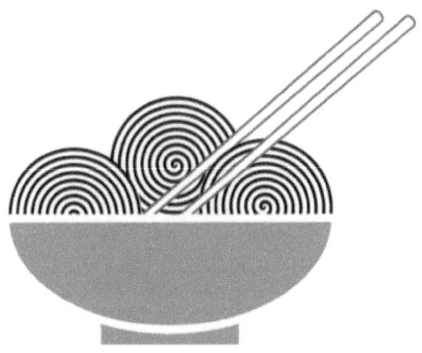

I'm just someone who likes cooking and for whom sharing food is a form of expression.

- Maya Angelou

Epilogue

Voilà! You have practised self-love by taking time to pause and ponder about your lifestyle and state of health.

Every day, you live a healthier life when you set your mind to it and take appropriate actions. How do you feel after spending quiet time to work toward your health and fitness goals? Pen your thoughts in this section and prosper.

You are now ready to take concrete steps and real actions towards your health and fitness goals. Remember, obstacles are part of the way.

May you become the healthier version of yourself that you have set out to become.

_____

_____

_____

_____

_____

_____

Abbreviation

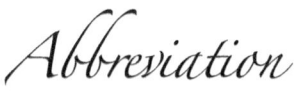

ml	millilitre
L	litre
g	gramme
kg	kilogramme
tsp	teaspoon
tbs	tablespoon
min.	minute

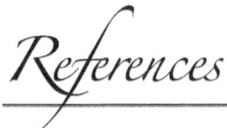

References

American Heart Association, https://www.heart.org, last accessed July 2020.

BBC Good Food, https://www.bbcgoodfood.com, last accessed July 2020.

Beijing Tong Ren Tang, https://cm.tongrentang.com/en/article/367.html, last accessed July 2020.

Bell, A. (2020), *Plant Power: Protein-Rich Recipes for Vegetarians and Vegans* (Hachette: UK).

Bloomsbury Publishing (2017), *Super Food: Beetroot* (Bloomsbury Publishing: UK).

Bloomsbury Publishing (2017), *Super Food: Cucumber* (Bloomsbury Publishing: UK).

Bloomsbury Publishing (2017), *Super Food: Lemon* (Bloomsbury Publishing: UK).

Diniz, R. (2012), *A Woman's Guide to Sensible Eating* (Broadway Publishing House: India).

DK (2017), *Sprouted!: Seeds, Grains and Beans—Power Up Your Plate with Home-Sprouted Superfoods* (Dorling Kindersley: UK).

DK (2017), *How Food Works: The Facts Visually Explained* (Dorling Kindersley: UK).

DK (2017), *The Science of Cooking: Every Question Answered to Give You the Edge* (Dorling Kindersley: UK).

Fulton, M. (1993), *New Cookbook: Cooking for Family and Friends* (Cornstalk Publishing: Australia).

Griffiths, C., and Valsamis, V. (2017), *The Vegetable: Recipes That Celebrate Nature* (Smith Street Books: Australia).

Harvard Medical, Harvard Health Publishing, https://www.health.harvard.edu, last accessed July 2020.

Institute for Functional Medicine, https://www.ifm.org, last accessed July 2020.

Klenerman, P. (2017), *The Immune System: A Very Short Introduction* (Oxford University Press).

Lin Qianliang and Chen Xiaoyi (2014), *Tea Therapy: Natural Remedies Using Traditional Chinese Medicine* (Shanghai Press and Publishing Development Company / Better Link Press).

Low, E. (2015), *The Little Teochew Cookbook* (Marshall Cavendish: Singapore).

Mangini, C. (2015), *The Vegetable Butcher: How to Select, Prep, Slice, Dice, and Masterfully Cook Vegetables from Artichokes to Zucchini.*

Mayo Clinic, https://www.mayoclinic.org, last accessed August 2020.

McIntyre, A. (2016), *Healing Drinks: Delicious Recipes for Body and Mind (100 Healthy Recipes)* (Bounty Books: UK).

Medical News Today, https://www.medicalnewstoday.com/, last accessed July 2020.

Medicine Net, https://www.medicinenet.com/script/main/hp.asp, last accessed July 2020.

Mind Body Green, https://www.mindbodygreen.com, last accessed July 2020.

Mindful magazine, www.mindful.org, last accessed July 2020.

Morgan, S. (2012), *Party Nuts!: 50 Recipes for Spicy, Sweet, Savoury, and Simply Sensational Nuts That Will Be the Hit of Any Gathering* (Harvard Common Press: USA).

National Geographic (2017), *Natural Home Remedies: Easy Ways to Feel Better, Live Longer and Enrich Your Life*, National Geographic (USA).

Pinnock, D. (2018), *Eat Your Way to a Healthy Heart: Tackle Heart Disease by Changing the Way You Eat, in 50 Recipes (The Medicinal Chef)* (Quadrille Publishing: UK).

Prevention magazine, https://www.prevention.com, last accessed July 2020.

Real Simple, https://www.realsimple.com, last accessed August 2020.

South China Morning Post, https://www.scmp.com/lifestyle/food-drink, last accessed 16 August 2020.

Tan, C. (2004), *The Family Herbal Cookbook* (Times Edition: Singapore).

Tan, T. (2007), *Naturally Speaking: Chinese Recipes and Home Remedies* (Marshall Cavendish: Singapore).

Time magazine, https://time.com/longform/food-best-medicine/, last accessed July 2020.

The Australian Women's Weekly (2008), *Salad Days* (ACP Books: Australia).

The Australian Women's Weekly (2008), *The Essential Soup Cookbook* (ACP Books: Australia).

The Center for Mindful Eating, https://thecenterformindful eating.org, last accessed July 2020.

The Mindful Kitchen (2020), *Confessions of a Terrible Cook* (Lion's Roar Special Publication: USA).

WebMD, https://www.webmd.com/, last accessed July 2020.

World Health Organisation, https://www.who.int/news-room/fact-sheets/detail/food-safety, last accessed July 2020.

Worndl, B. (2018), *Fruit: Recipes That Celebrate Nature* (Smith Street Books: Australia).

The body is your temple.
Keep it pure and clean for
the soul to reside in.
- B. K. S. Iyengar

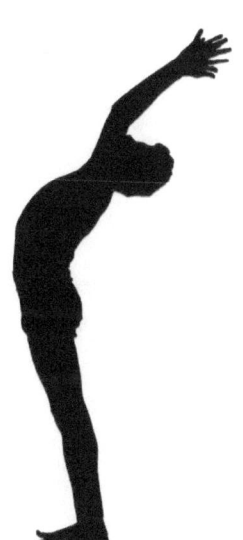

About the Author

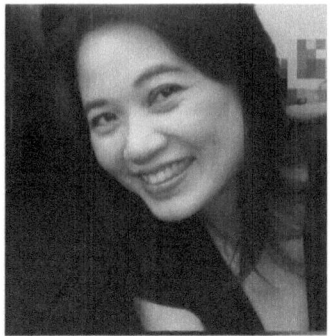

Louise YT Phua is a talent coach for global citizens and international nomads in life and work transitions. Louise thrives in people development. Together with her clients, she helps individuals and organisations to construct and realise their future selves.

In her practice as a talent coach / facilitator of adult learning, Louise encounters many adults who have struggled with health issues. The majority of Louise's coaching clients and learners are urbanites in their twenties, thirties, forties, and fifties. Often, these clients are deeply engrossed in career progression that they have forgotten that *health is wealth*. When health checks and nagging aches reveal serious conditions, these adult learners look for instant gratification and quick fixes.

When Louise published her first booklet, *Myrita*, in 2019, she received overwhelming encouragement from friends, family, and peers. *Myrita* is inspired by the Spanish name Rita, which means 'pearl'. *Myrita* is a space to pause, ponder, and prosper about life projects and new priorities. This series of booklets is designed to help readers explore, experiment, and expand their lives, therefore finding their own pearls of wisdom.

Louise has almost twenty years' work experience in talent acquisition and people development. On a daily basis, Louise interacts with a wide spectrum of talents with various professions, nationalities, personalities, and aspirations. As she specialises in the life science and consumer markets, a majority of the talents that Louise works with include dentists, doctors, flavourists, food scientists, food technologists, healthcare economists, hospital administrators, logisticians, microbiologists, nutritionists, packaging professionals, pharmacists, consumer marketing specialists, etc. During her conversations with these talents, they exchange knowledge about various aspects of life science.

A Singaporean by birth, she has worked and lived in Australia, China, France, and Malaysia. While effectively bilingual in English and Chinese, Louise also speaks basic French and Bahasa Indonesia. She is a serious practitioner of mindfulness and Iyengar yoga.

Louise holds a MA Lifelong Learning from University College London Institute of Education and a BA Marketing and the Media from Murdoch University, Western Australia. A certified coach in positive psychology, Louise has completed a Harvard certificate in six-week plan for healthy eating.

A self-declared bland food queen, Louise's Teochew's family lives on a diet with low sugar, low salt, and little oil. Louise favours the natural taste of fresh produce.

At the heart of it, Louise relishes the personal story of how each earthling overcomes obstacles and becomes slightly better version of oneself.

www.ingramcontent.com/pod-product-compliance
Lightning Source LLC
Chambersburg PA
CBHW032028290526
45786CB00011B/1144